THE NUANCES

IN NAVIGAING MEDICAL SCHOOL

A STRATEGIC GUIDE TO MANAGING PROBLEMS FACED ON THE PATH TO BECOMING A PHYSICIAN

LEIZA O'NEIL

ISBN 978-1-7366278-1-5

This book is dedicated to everyone who has supported me through the years, and to my students ...past, present, and future.

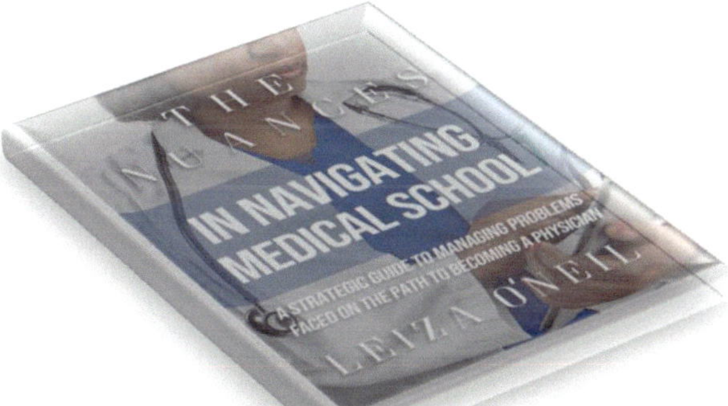

Contents

ACKNOWLEDGMENTS

When I think about individuals I would like to acknowledge upon completion of this book, my immediate family comes to mind. If I were to list each name, the list would be between twenty-five to thirty individuals. Each one of them have extended their love and support to me in one way or another. I am so lucky to have them all.

I would however like to specially mention my mom whose prayers have kept me to this very moment. Mom, I love you with all my heart.

My two younger sisters, Jahn and Oreisa, have kept me to task and has been a constant reminder to me of what I can accomplish. Even though you are my younger sisters I look up to both of you.

For the gentle nudges from my niece Arienne and my sister Esther, I love you completely.

To my friends Gail and Mel (Edrene), by telling me about and helping me find myself you give me my voice. Thanks for the many hours we spent on the phone.

To my tech buddy Bryant, you have never let me down and I have always been able to count on you from the day we met.

To my personal cheerleader Ron, you believe in me more than I believe in myself.

The encouragement from each and every individual who extended themselves is what helped me take each step towards the completion of this book. For that, I say thank you from the bottom of my heart. I love and appreciate you all.

Most of all, I thank God for the journey. He has brought me through the process of writing this book. We have gone from Him putting on my heart to share my experience with a larger audience, for which I dumbed it down as just wanting to share a few PowerPoint slides, to Him placing the opportunity before me to be a presenter at a conference for which I reluctantly accepted. It has been seven years since He first gave me the idea to write this book. He has patiently dragged His stubborn child to the finish line. In the process, endless tears have been shed, and an abundance of grace and mercy have been extended. I have been molded and changed. I am certainly not where I should be but thank God I am not where I was. Most of all I thank Him for stretching me beyond what I thought was possible. As I move forward, my goal will always be to help others, even if it is just one person, take a step forward.

INTRODUCTION

Welcome to 'The Nuances of Navigating Medical School'! This book seeks to give you guidance with the rarely discussed but frequent occurrences that can derail your medical school career. The goal is to help you navigate, avoid, or appropriately deal with rare but possible issues that may arise. Whether you are looking forward to beginning or are newly in residency, there are chapters in this book that will assist you in knowing what you can expect and present you with options for resolve.

There are things that every fourth year medical student can tell a first year student that they wish *they* had known when they began. It is those little titbits of information that can make a big difference in your medical school journey. It can determine how you manage your time, where you put your emphasis and how you make crucial choices. Missteps in medical school can be both financially and emotionally costly. No one wants to be the one saying, *"If I'd known…"*.

Along the four year journey; there will be times when issues will develop from out of nowhere and having an idea of what both your choices and resources are as you go about resolving those issues will make all the difference in the world. Keep in mind; -this is not the kind of book that will give you answers to every issue that arises in medical school. It will, however, give you options for solving some of those issues in a manner that is best suited for you. Medical school is not 'one size fits all'; making choices that allow you to go through the process with the least amount of stress will be immensely helpful.

The ultimate goal of a medical student is to match into a residency program. It is a goal that is becoming more and more challenging as the number of medical students entering the match increases, while available positions stay the same or increase at a non-compatible rate. However, if you go into the process prepared and knowledgeable, you will increase your chances of NOT being washed out in the SOAP *(Supplemental Offer and*

Acceptance Program). At this point, first and second-year students tend to have no idea what the SOAP is and third and fourth-year students have only heard that it is to be avoided at all costs. This is because as you enter medical school, the rate of information coming at you is such that if you do not have excellent time management skills, you will rarely have time to think about anything else but the next test. If you plot your journey carefully, before entering or at least at the beginning of your first year and learn to avoid pitfalls by being familiar with the process, you can plot a course that will lead in the opposite direction of "soaping". Giving you valuable knowledge to plotting a successful course is what this book will help you do.

Being knowledgeable about what choices to make and being happier throughout the process is the goal. My belief is that happy doctors, save lives, literally and figuratively. On the other hand, unhappy doctors can cost lives, literally and figuratively. My goal has always been to make sure medical students are happier with both the process and their specialty choice, leading to doctors that are happier overall.

Providing vital information will aid in preparing you for the journey you are about to embark on. So, join me as we seek to tackle the challenges of medical school together.

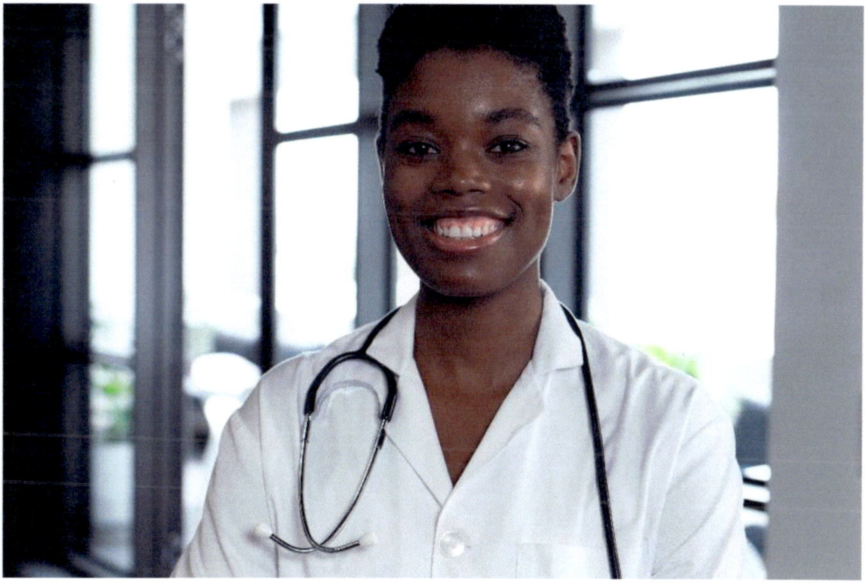

1

WHAT YOU SHOULD KNOW BEFORE STARTING MEDICAL SCHOOL

Before starting medical school, you should be aware of the fact that you are about to begin a journey unlike any other. Of course, the best way to get through any journey is to be prepared. In the process of preparing, you will first need to adjust your expectations. You should know that in medical school the volume of information you will have to learn in the first week is not even close to being like your first month of undergrad. The biggest mistakes new students make is thinking that they can do what they did in undergrad for medical school. Most times the volume of information is too much to process in the same way, and the faster you can make the adjustment the better it will be for you.

The experience is also very different for each individual. For some the journey will be easy and for others it will be hard but there is really no other experience that is as rewarding. It is unlike any other journey you have encountered, and you will not always be able to rely on family and friends to understand. Even though *you* may have a family member that is a physician, what *you* go through today may be very different from what *they* went through a few years ago.

Year one. Again, there will be a *large* volume of information you will be responsible for learning. Not just memorizing but learning. Know the difference. Why? Because you will see this information again and if you didn't learn it the first time you will have to spend valuable time re-learning the material. Understand you will already be required to put in twice as much time studying as you did in undergrad. And just when you think youv'e pushed yourself to the limit and can not go any further summer arrives. *Hallelujah!?!?* No.

Many are fooled into thinking that because it's summer, they can rest and relax until school starts back in the fall. That's a classic mistake. Why? Your CV! When applying for residencies three years later the question will come up 'What did you do during the summer of your first year in medical school?' You will need to show that you were productive; so find a doctor to shadow, a research project to work on or something medically related to do. You will need these activities to show on your CV and ERAS application. Consider it valuable prep work for the ultimate goal, - 'getting into residency'.

Year two. You will be required to process the same volume of work you did in year one with additional responsibilities. For example whereas you may not have had to do NBME exams in year one, you may be required to do them in year two. Now you are required to do much more with the same amount of time. This is where some students fall into trouble. You will need to get organized and manage your time wisely. You will no longer have time for that social life you've been cultivating all of undergrad. This will increase the time you spend with classmates who are going through the same things you are. If you didn't make connections in year one you may find yourself isolated. *Do Not Isolate Yourself.* Schedule time to attend social events held by the class and get involved. These are 'get to know you' events with your classmates, and this bonding time will come in handy when placed in teams to rotate in the hospital later on.

The summer of year two you'll most likely be studying for Step 1. Do not make plans that will have you rushing to take the test, and in turn, jeopardize your score. You may not understand now but Step 1 is SUPER important.

Year three. At this point you may feel like you've maximized your time and learning potential but keep in mind: that you will have to do everything you did in the first and second year but in year three you'll have to add seeing patients and rounding in the hospital to the mix. This is where you are going to peak in how well you manage your time getting required tasks done and studying for your medical shelves and other exams. You've got to get that together quickly because this year will also test your strength to endure. Just as you may have gotten use to balancing all the extra stuff thrown your way ERAS comes along and upsets your schedule. 'I can't' are usually the first words that may come to mind but consider all you have gone through and the fact that you want and need to match to pay back those loans! Then you must quickly kick into gear and find a way to get it done. And don't forget you now have Step 2 on your plate, both CS (Clinical Skills) and CK (Clinical Knowledge). You'll certainly feel like there are not enough hours in the day!

(As of 2020 the Clinical Skills test has been canceled and is no longer a requirement.)

Year four. If you've planned your schedule right, this is your cooling off year. You will be traveling because of interviews, and some rotations will be a little lighter in terms of responsibility because you will have the third-year students to fill in the gap. This is when you have the freedom to take some time to reconnect with friends and family, catch up on sleep, and check things off your *med-bucket list* before residency. You will be able to enjoy the festivities of match week and graduation IF you planned right and were prepared.

Keep in mind that as challenging as medical school may be, it is equally as rewarding. You will meet people and be exposed to cultures from all over the country and yes, the world. You will bond and create lifelong friendships. If helping others bring you joy, you will never *work a day* in your life although your body may at times disagree with you. There will be many days ahead when you will look back and know that it was worth it.

(This is another activity that the year 2020 has affected for medical students. Because of COVID-19 interviews are now done online and away rotations are limited.)

2

FIRST YEAR OF MEDICAL SCHOOL

What to expect

Having planned nearly a dozen freshman orientations. It is always so exhilarating to see the new, bright-eyed, and energetic faces of students that are so excited to have arrived in medical school. I tend to encourage that excitement because I believe in soaking in the good moments in life. But just one short week after the conclusion of freshman orientation there is always a stark difference. The first week of classes has ended, the energy has changed 180 degrees, and it can be seen on each face. Every member of the incoming class can then be placed in one of three groups:

- Group one: Students are cautiously confident and know that they are going to have to work hard. So, they talk to upper classmen and try to get prepared so they can get it done.

- Group two: Students tend to pair themselves with one or two like-minded classmates and decide 'we can do this together'.
- Group three: These students are the most vulnerable. They get scared and do one of two things. (a.) they isolate themselves or (b.) they seek help reaching out to administrators and professors, not quite knowing what they are seeking help for.

Now there are exceptions to every rule, so occasionally you will find "gunners" in the class who are overly confident, or "saboteurs" who think bringing others down will help them rise. Stay away from them. They are the students who usually receive the biggest reality check by the first exam.

Now you may be thinking 'which group should I aim to be in?' The truth is you should aim to be in all three. First, take the time to speak to upper classmen and find out the pitfalls and what to expect. Every school is different.

Then, associate yourself with one or two other like-minded classmates. It's just easier to go through this process with the support of others who are going through the same things. And finally, know that it is okay to be scared. You are starting a new journey and if there aren't a few butterflies in your stomach, something is wrong. Be confident of the fact that you have been accepted to medical school. Many people have done it before, and you will be able to do it also. Keep in mind there will be times that you will need to isolate yourself so you can get yourself together to be a productive member of a group. Your schedule may not be your friends' schedule; the way you study may not be the way your friends' study, so know when to pull back. If you can't figure it out seek help by making a list of what you are having trouble with and find an advisor to talk with. Do not walk into someone's office expecting them to give you a magic answer to everything. That answer does not exist. Be specific about what you need, so you can *get* the specific help you need.

Tips for the first year

In medical school, the most-free time you will have is in your first year.

- ***TIP:*** Learn to manage your time.

You don't have very much time to adjust after the reality check of how much information you will be responsible for learning. The faster you can adjust the better. Create a schedule, get organized, and be realistic about what you will need to accomplish. This will be an asset in the years to come.

You are now in the business of learning. If you have never tapped into your organizational and management skills before, do it NOW.

- ***TIP:*** Figure out how you learn.

There are seven learning styles. Know which one fits you, or which combination fits you best and then study the material in your learning style. The last thing you want to do is spend twice the time studying the way everyone *else* is studying and not get the desired results. This hits your self-esteem hard because you start thinking that you are not as good as others. Such thinking is a mistake that takes too much time and energy to bounce back from. It can sometimes end your medical school career before it takes off. Save yourself the drama; figure out how you learn; focus on you.

Again, medical school is a place where the sheer volume of material you will need to learn can take you out.

- ***TIP:*** Find an app or a class and learn how to speed-read.

Doing this before starting medical school would work best. This is certainly the time when it is going to be an asset. Speed reading is not just about going through the information faster; it is also about comprehending faster. The more information you can comprehend the first time you go through it, the shorter your review sessions will be. Take the time to do this the first year because you will not have the time in the following years when it will be most needed.

Knowing what's ahead helps you to get focused.

- ***TIP:*** Go to the AAMC or the Careers in Medicine websites and get familiar with what you should be accomplishing each year of medical school towards your goal of residency.

Keep track of what you should be doing each year, put it on your schedule or calendar, and keep focused; it will lessen the chances of you falling behind. You do not want to fall behind because catching up can be an energy drainer.

- ***TIP:*** Take advantage of assessments.

Assessments will give you focus and direction as you progress through medical school; having direction will help with the decisions and choices you are faced with later on. Take advantage of the information on those websites previously mentioned.

WARNING: Do not focus on a single specialty from year one.

- ***TIP:*** Have an idea of what kind of medicine you will want to practice. Narrow it down to your top three specialties.

I know you've always wanted to be a surgeon. Everything on your Curriculum Vitae says surgery, but I can't tell you how many times students focus from year one on a specialty, then get to third year rotations and fall in love with another specialty. Diversify. Shadow physicians, especially in areas of interest. Also, it is important to shadow and complete rotations in areas that are not offered at your institution, such as the subspecialties. My advice is to choose three specialties that pique your interest and get to know them. If you find one you absolutely do not like, replace it with another. By third year one of the choices on your list should stand out, giving you a top specialty choice. This advice will be especially relevant if your *Step 1* score falls short of where it needs to be.

Here is a short story about this tip. I had a student who walked into medical school, and from day one declared that he was going to be a surgeon. Everything he did from that point was driven by his surgery dreams. He did well in his first and second year, but then he stumbled on Step 1 and did not receive a surgery competitive score. He tried to bounce back by attempting to get a really good Step 2 CK score but also fell short. When ERAS came around, he decided to apply for surgery knowing that he was not competitive. Although he was advised to apply to a second specialty, he decided to apply to only surgery. He applied to over eighty programs. He got about five interviews. Match Week he discovered he did not match. He was devastated. He entered what we now call the SOAP process. Back then it was called the Scramble. He scrambled into an internal medicine position but was not happy about it. We had a talk; I told him that he would need to change his perspective and attitude in order to be successful in that residency. We talked long and hard about the meaning of life and what was important to him. He thanked me for helping him to feel better and left my office. After graduation later that year I never saw or heard from him again. Seven years later, I'm sitting at my desk, and I get a call. On that call I discovered that the student had gone on and finished the internal medicine residency. That morning he had a ribbon-cutting to open his first dialysis center. Once he had a quiet moment in his office, he remembered our conversation from years earlier, found my number, and called me to thank me for changing his perspective and consequently, his life. As an internal medicine physician, he is both a successful doctor and business owner. Keep your options open!

Mentorship is key.

- ***Tip:*** Find mentors in every area possible and stay connected.

I tend to advise medical students to treat their medical school career like the presidency. Form a cabinet of mentors and keep them close. You should have two second year mentors; have at least one mentor each from the third and fourth year, have a basic science faculty mentor, and a clinical science faculty mentor. Also, have an administrator on your cabinet that you can call on if needed. If you surround yourself with individuals that can advise you, the process of rising quickly when you fall into trouble will be less painful. Your clinical mentors will also come in handy at the end of year three when you will need letters of recommendation for your residency application.

Helping Loved Ones Understand

As you begin to understand just how much of your time and effort medical school requires, it will become increasingly clear that there will be birthdays, anniversaries and even weddings you will not be able to attend. Now, birthdays and anniversaries do not change from year to year so pre-plan and try to fit them in your schedule way in advance. If there is a conflict (eg. an exam), explain and decline well in advance. It is important to avoid unnecessary distractions before exams.

Due to the substantial amount of time you will spend studying and on rotations, you will need to help husbands, wives and other family members understand this by giving them access to your schedule. Make good use of the time when you are not in school and are spending time with them. It is always best to help when you can; and do not create extra chores for them. If loved ones are away from you, pre-plan activities for when they or you visit. If they see you making an effort, and are aware of how hectic your schedule is, they will be more apt to understand. Do your best to forewarn spouses of upcoming changes.

For some of you, there may be tough issues and choices to deal with that are out of your control. A loved one going through sickness or a death, which can be especially tough when dealing with the pressures of medical school, can make you feel twice as bad. When family members look to you for guidance in such issues, remember delegating what needs to be done is your best form of leadership.

3

SECOND YEAR

It's all about Step 1

As you begin your second year, the first and second month will be about adjusting to the new volume. Right after that, Step 1 will begin to become more of a reality. The more you think about it, the more nervous you may begin to feel. Putting it out of your mind and just waiting to cram at the end of the year is one way to deal with it, and although it has worked for some in past years, there is another option.

Try as you may, the thought of Step 1 is going to keep resurfacing throughout second year. So, here's an option for dealing with that. As December of second year approaches you have now completed two thirds of the information needed for Step 1.

- On your December break take a full practice exam

for Step 1. You are not taking it expecting a great passing score. You are taking it to get an idea of where your base line is. That means 'how much of the information needed for Step 1 do I have in my head without studying?' When you take the baseline test without studying and you get a score, that is your base line number. That is the number you're going to start climbing from. You can now use that number to determine what kind of study schedule you need to build. Will you need to put in a lot of study time, or will you be able to carefully pace yourself?

- The next thing you should pay attention to from the results of the practice test are the areas that tell you how you did in specific subjects. Look at where you are weakest and start by studying that subject matter or those subject matters first. After doing about a month of specific studying, take another practice test. Your score should have jumped at least ten points. If it hasn't, you may not be studying in a manner that is best for you. Figure out how you learn and amend your study method ASAP.

By starting the studying process for Step 1 in this way, you have done three very important things:

- You're knowledgeable about where you are, how far you need to go, and you have an idea of how much study time you'll need to put in to get there.
- You can now determine the effectiveness of your studying. Knowing that this early, gives you time to make changes before the test.
- You will also know what areas you should spend the most time on and which areas you can be confident in.

Isn't studying for Step 1 with focused information much better than studying everything in sight hoping to get a passing score?

What if I didn't get a good score?

If you did not get a good score, try hard to let it go. That's easier said than done. I know. But there are more productive ways to spend your time than pining over a low score. First, assess what went wrong, so you can make changes before Step 2 CK. Second, you should treat every patient you see during the third year as if they are a question on an exam. Third, start your study schedule early, and try to get through your study material more than once. And forth, decide if you need extra study help -such as a study aide- and add it to your schedule sooner rather than later. Gage your progress along the way, and set a goal that will enable you to 'beast the next test', Step 2 CK.

Do not get stuck thinking *'I studied so hard for Step 1 and didn't get the result I wanted. What am I going to do for Step 2?'* That is unproductive thinking. You are fully engaged in a life of test taking now. Figure out what went wrong and fix it. Step 2 is around the corner and Step 3 will be here before you know it. Do not waste time at the pity party. Do whatever you can to fix it and slay it:

- Figure out how you learn best.
- TAKE TIME to learn to speed read/comprehend.
- Get a study aide.
- Give yourself enough time to study.
- Find a study partner if necessary.
- Ask for help.
- Organize your schedule.
- Manage your time.

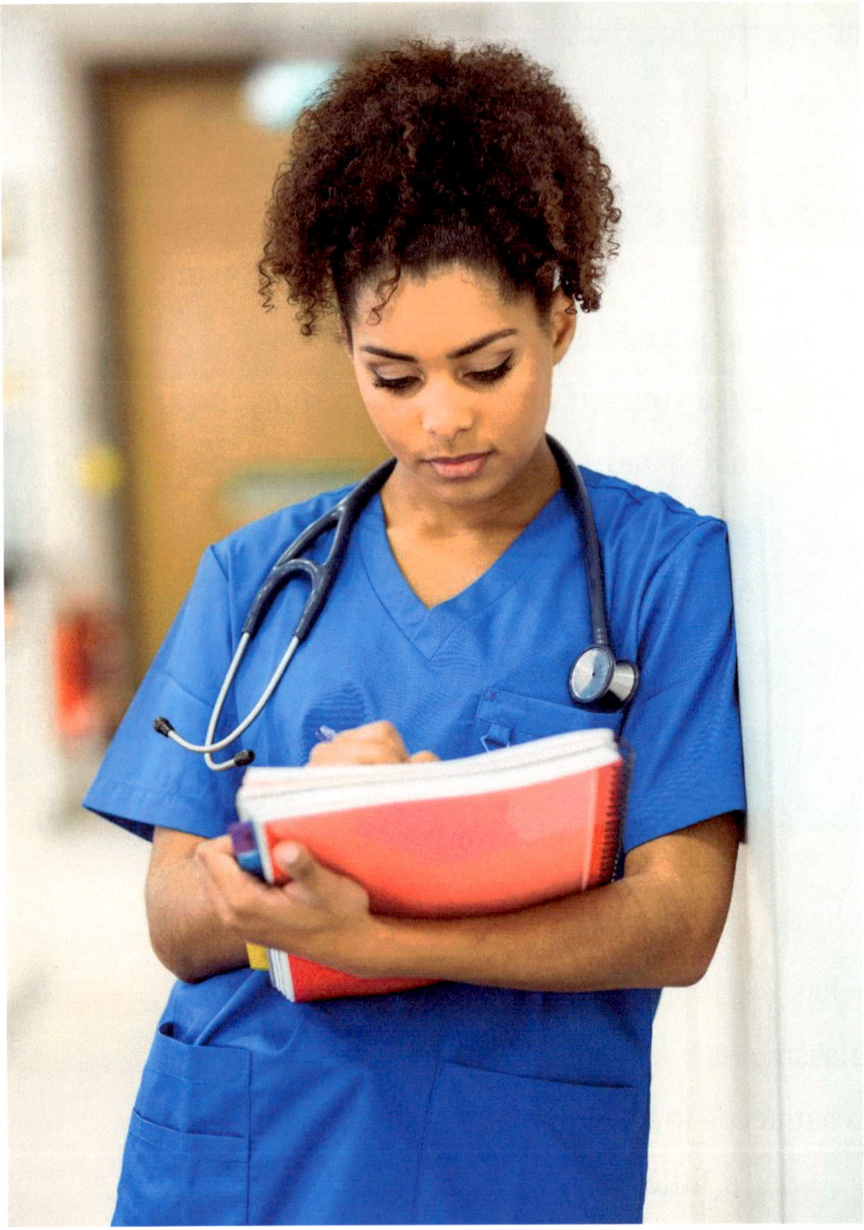

4

THIRD YEAR

What should I be doing?

This is the most difficult year of medical school. While adjusting to your third-year schedule you are forced to do planning for your fourth year. There is so much to do that some students choose to bury their heads in the sand and hope that their list will magically be complete when they come up for air. That is not going to happen and delaying the inevitable just makes it worse. The earlier you start the better.

My suggestion is to sit down with someone who knows what fourth year entails. This is when those upper classmen mentors will come in rather handy. Get a list of what needs to be done and schedule it by due dates so that you get a little done every month for third year. Just by getting students organized for this process, you have no idea how many lives I'm told I save this time of year, even though I'm not a doctor.

Also, keep in mind that none of the following will matter if you fail a shelf. So most importantly, keep studying and passing your shelves (NBME's).

This will be different for every institution but here is an idea of how things run at the institution I am familiar with.

- Aug-Oct – get adjusted to your third-year schedule. Decide what specialty you will pursue. Start a running list of who you will ask for letters of recommendation (LoR). You should have someone you can ask for a LoR after each rotation.
- Nov – During Thanksgiving break work on your CV. Bullet-point some ideas for your personal statement. Get a group together to start practicing for Step 2 CS.
- Dec – Work on your personal statement. Research programs in your specialty. Start making a list of

programs you will apply to. Take a CK practice test. Create a study schedule.

- ☐ Jan – Decide where you would like to apply for VSAS. Work on getting your documents together for the process. Know the date programs begin accepting applications.
- ☐ Feb – Start working on your fourth-year schedule. Time to focus on getting dates for CS and CK.
- ☐ Mar – Talk to fourth-year students about the Match process. Start finalizing the list of programs you want to apply to.
- ☐ Apr – ERAS is now available for LoR's to be uploaded. Request your letters.
- ☐ May – Meet with your advisor about your MSPE (Medical Student Performance Evaluation). This is a good time to sit for Step 2 CS.
- ☐ Jun – Track down LoR writers before they leave for vacation. This is the month you should be finalizing your CV and personal statement. Get them completed so you can focus on other important things in the coming months.

- ☐ Jul – Focus on finishing your ERAS application. You should have sat for at least one of your Steps by now. This is a good time to sit for Step 2 CK.
- ☐ Aug - Check and recheck that you have completed everything for ERAS. Then review, have others review, and re-review to make sure there are no mistakes, and that you are ready for submission.
- ☐ Sept – Make sure you have uploaded a *professional* picture. Submit ERAS.

Congratulations!!! You finally have your life back. You have done all this while studying, taking shelves, managing patients and preparing for Steps.

Planning your Fourth Year Schedule

In planning your fourth-year schedule the first step, is to know what you want, and what will make you happy. What does that have to do with scheduling? Everything. If you know where you are going it's easier to plan how to get there. That is the whole point of this book. It is no different when planning the rest of your life.

Some of the decisions you will have to make are:

- What specialty do I want to practice?
- Where in the country do I want to work?
- What are the programs in that area?
- Which ones will I apply to for VSAS?
- Do I want to do an international elective?

Once you have considered and have answered these questions, the next thing you will need to work on is timing.

Fact is that the fourth-year schedule is not a one-size-fits-all. You will need to keep in mind the nuances of your chosen specialty when planning your schedule.

Here are some things to consider:

August – Most students tend to take this month off to study for and take Step 2 CK. But, if, for example, you are doing Surgery, Orthopedics or Emergency Medicine, you will want to plan for and schedule doing Step 2 CK earlier; you will want to spend the month of August doing an away rotation. Doing away rotations for these specialties are helpful to the Match process. You will want to get them done early so that you can also acquire a Letter of Recommendation or Student Letter of Evaluation.

My August Rotation is:______________________________

September – This is the month that the ERAS application should be submitted. I know that there is no hard-due date for the application, but with as many applicants as there are, *earlier* certainly is better. Remember ERAS opens September 15th at 9 AM.

My September Rotation is:___________________________

October – October is the month for the Medical Student Performance Evaluation (MSPE) to be submitted. Based on my experience there are some specialties like Internal Medicine and Pediatrics that give interview invites before the MSPE is released. The exceptions to this are the ROADS specialties. (Radiology, Orthopedics, Anesthesiology, Dermatology and Surgery), which tend to wait until after MSPE to begin sending out invites. Once the MSPE is released however, all specialties begin to send out invites.

My October Rotation is:______________________________

November – This is the month when you should assess. How many interviews do I have? Will I be able to make them all? Which ones will I consider canceling? If I do not have enough, should I begin contacting programs to show interest? Should I have a talk with my advisor? Should I begin reaching out to alumni who may be at my programs of interest?

My November Rotation is:______________________________

December – This is the first month in medical school when relaxing *may* be an option. It is only if you have planned your schedule right and manage to schedule a lighter rotation that this could be possible. Take the time to look at all the institutions where you have interviewed and take notes. If you have used the AAMC app (The Match Prism), this will be easier for you. It allows you to input the programs where you are interviewing, rate them, and make notes about the experience.

My December Rotation is:______________________________

January – This month you will do your last interviews and start putting together your rank list. This is when your nerves will start to do overtime but settle yourself and focus on what you want for your life as you create your rank list.

My January Rotation is:________________________________

February – The rank list is due. There is nothing left to be said. Finding a rotation to keep you occupied so that there is less time to sit and ponder may be best. I tend to say that it is now up to faith/fate - whichever you may believe in.

My February Rotation is:_______________________________

March – Match Day is here. Keep in mind that if there is a ceremony, family may be coming to town. Do not forget that there may be airport or bus depot pickups required, but by now you have the best-ever organizational and time management skills. You will want time to celebrate with friends and family. There are hair and nails to be done, outfits to buy. It is a celebratory month. Everyone celebrates differently. Choose a rotation that will be in line with your activities for the month.

My March Rotation is:_________________________________

April - By April celebrating has taken its toll. You now know where in the country you will reside. If you have not taken your month off yet, this will be the best time to do so. You can take time to look for a place, relocate, and maybe even do some traveling. If you have taken your month off before now, a rotation that will also allow you to have weekends free to do these things should be considered.

My April Rotation is:______________________________

Congratulations!! Your fourth-year schedule is complete, and preparation for graduation is next. Of course, there is a list of things that must be checked off for graduation, so be sure to complete everything. You've come too far to drop the ball now.

Away Rotations

The most popular question about away rotations is 'how do I choose my away rotation?' Here is the method I suggest to students who have no idea where to begin. I ask, ‘what would make you happiest, working in a hot or cold climate?’ That answer cuts the continent in half horizontally. Then I ask, ‘would you rather the east coast or west coast?’ That answer cut it in half vertically. Now take the quadrant of the US that you have chosen and make a list of every program in your specialty choice. Once you have gotten your list, start comparing programs. A good place to start is AMA’s FREIDA online. On that site there is a chart that allows you to compare programs side by side. This feature can be very helpful in comparing salary, duty hours, the mean step scores etcetera. Once you have prioritized your list, apply to your choice institutions. If you are planning to do only one away rotation, apply to two. Apply to four if you are planning to do two rotations. That way you can insure getting your dates, and if one falls through, you won’t fall apart.

If by chance you are applying bi-coastal, I suggest that you set up all your away rotations on one coast first, and then the other. Try to use your rotations as an audition, so that you are offered an interview before leaving.

Please consider this. Since stats differ from institution to institution, you may want to poll the fourth-year students ahead of you to find out how many of them match to an institution where they did an away rotation. The stats at my institution are very low for students matching where they did away rotations. I have not been able to put a solid finger on a reason for it, but it is something you may want to consider.

CV Advice

CAUTION: the advice given here you probably won't get from any other Student Affairs administrator or Dean.

I know you are told that a curriculum vita should have everything you have ever done on it and it should be detailed. But if you were a program director going through hundreds, maybe even thousands of CV's, what would you want to see? The time a student worked at Chick-fil-a or pertinent information such as their shadowing or research experience?

Because you are creating a CV in the beginning stages of your career, it should look like that. This document will follow you for the rest of your medical career. A proper beginning will enable you to keep it as a living document that you can simply add to as the years go by.

If you had another career that is not medically related before you began medical school, listing two or three pages of what is considered non-relevant stuff before getting to your medical experiences will very rarely benefit you in this process, and can do more harm than good. I know… I know… a CV should have *everything*, but do you want to be right or matched?

Instead create a medical career CV. Start by making a list of everything you have done that is relevant. Because it is also an academic document, don't forget to include tutoring and teaching experiences. All research experience should also be included. Your past career items should be listed with dates, but do not go into details.

How do you decide which details are important and which are not? Here's an example that I tend to use. Let's say you worked one summer in college as a lifeguard, and another working at McDonalds. I would list McDonalds as a line item with the appropriate date. However, because working as a lifeguard has clinically related experience, I would be more detailed. For example, you would need to be CPR certified to do life guarding, so I would list it.

When creating a CV, it should fit your career choice and the criteria of the employer. It should also be appropriate for the position. This should be your goal when putting together your document.

If you have a well put together CV, it should make filling out your ERAS application easier; it would be a matter of cutting and pasting. Your CV should be done in the middle of third year as previously suggested. That way you will be able to use it for both VSAS and ERAS. You can add additional items as you go.

Personal Statement Advice

Many times, students try to use their personal statement to impress, or get in the same mental space as a program director that has been in the field for years. I have also seen students pay quite a bit to have a professional write their personal statement. I can always tell, because when I read through it, I can just change the name and it would work for the next person… and the next… and the next. My point of view on this matter is that a personal statement should be personal. It should tell me a little about you, and what makes you unique and different from every other applicant.

I have read a lot of personal statements in the many years I have been in student affairs, but one has stayed with me over the years. I'll attempt to recap briefly. The student started by sharing that they had a habit of always holding their hands behind their back. As a child, people always noticed and commented about their long thin fingers. Because of that, the student became self-conscious and hid their hands behind their back. That is, until they started their surgery rotation. They realized that those long thin fingers had no problem doing things their classmates had trouble mastering. Surgery gave the one thing they thought was a flaw meaning and purpose, thus creating in them a passion. Now, this personal statement I'm referring to was just about a page in length, but I'll always remember it as 'the long thin fingers statement'. Even though admittedly I have a problem remembering names, I still remember *that* student's name years later. The reason I remember it is because the personal statement brought me a little closer to knowing that student intimately. It made me feel like I knew them after reading it. That should be your goal, to have the reader know a little bit more about you *the person* after reading your statement. It should not be a regurgitation of your CV.

Everyone will not have a story like that, but write about you, you are unique. Program directors will be able to pick you out of a crowd; believe me over 30,000 applicants is a *crowd*. This is your statement so make it count.

Here is a four-paragraph sample I give students to get them started:

Paragraph 1 - Why medicine? And don't tell me it's because you want to help people. There are several other professions you could have chosen that help people, so… *why medicine*?

Paragraph 2 – Now that you have gone through this gauntlet called medical school what have you learned about you? How have you become a better person equipped to serve others? *Why* do you still have a strong interest in medicine?

Paragraph 3 – What is your specialty choice; why?

Paragraph 4 – How do you intend to contribute globally?

Now look at those four paragraphs. Every individual will answer those questions differently. It's all about you. No cute quotes, anecdotes, or philosophical expressions about the specialty. It is a *personal* statement. Keep it personal and let the program director get a chance to know you.

Also, keep in mind that if you are applying to two specialties all you need to do is modify the third paragraph, not write a brand-new statement.

Choosing a Specialty

When students enter my office and tell me they can't decide on a specialty or that they like everything, I have no words of wisdom tucked in my pocket to give them. What I do is ask 'What rotations did you like best?' or 'What makes you happy?' Then I just sit back and watch their reaction when they answer the question. Nine out of ten times, the minute they mention the rotation that is 'the one' their face tells the story. They either light up or they smile. There is usually a reaction that is telling. When I point that out to them, then the excuses and reasons why not starts to flow. My response to that is to have them pull out a piece of paper and write down the pros and cons.

I know choosing a specialty is a big deal. It's so big; in fact, that the only consideration when making such a choice should be what makes you happy. Here's what I believe… 'Happy doctors save lives; unhappy doctors cost lives.' There are all sorts of things students take into consideration when choosing a specialty. The biggest one happens to be their Step 1 score.

CAUTION: Here is where *my* advice will differ from what you will hear from most advisors.

First, let me say I agree that your specialty choice should be in line with your step score. I also agree that your goals should be realistic. That's plan A. But through the years there have always been outlier's who have stepped out on *faith/fate* and gotten what they are passionate about, and not what they were qualified for. Every time I see that it just warms my heart to tears. Those individuals will be so much more effective in touching lives because they view being a doctor as an opportunity they have been given; it is not just a job. This goes two ways, -(a) students at the top of the class who can specialize in anything and choose primary care as their passion or (b) students who did not have the scores but got into specialties they were passionate about tend to become great doctors. They are passion driven.

I'm going to digress here and tell you a story. I had a student who came into my office feeling and looking so defeated; they didn't think their Step 1 score would make them competitive for the programs they wanted. I looked at the list of programs they applied to, and it was a list of community programs only. So, I told them a story. *(Yes, I tell many stories in my office. Just like 'there's an app for that', I've got a story for 'that'.)* I then asked them to do me a very expensive favor. I requested that they put four top Ivy League programs I suggested on their list. I'm sure they left my office thinking *'Ms. O'Neil's a little crazy'*, but they did it. They later interviewed at two of those four programs and matched at one of them. Of course, they had to make me tear up about it when they walked back into my office after match day and told me that even though I won't be there, every patient they see at that hospital will be an extension of me, because they wouldn't have been there if it wasn't for me. *OKAY…*, now back to the point. You never know what this universe has in store for your life. At least allow yourself the opportunity to be happy and give yourself a chance. Create a plan that is based on logic, but in addition, create a parallel plan and a dream plan also. But remember a longer list of programs *will not* guarantee success.

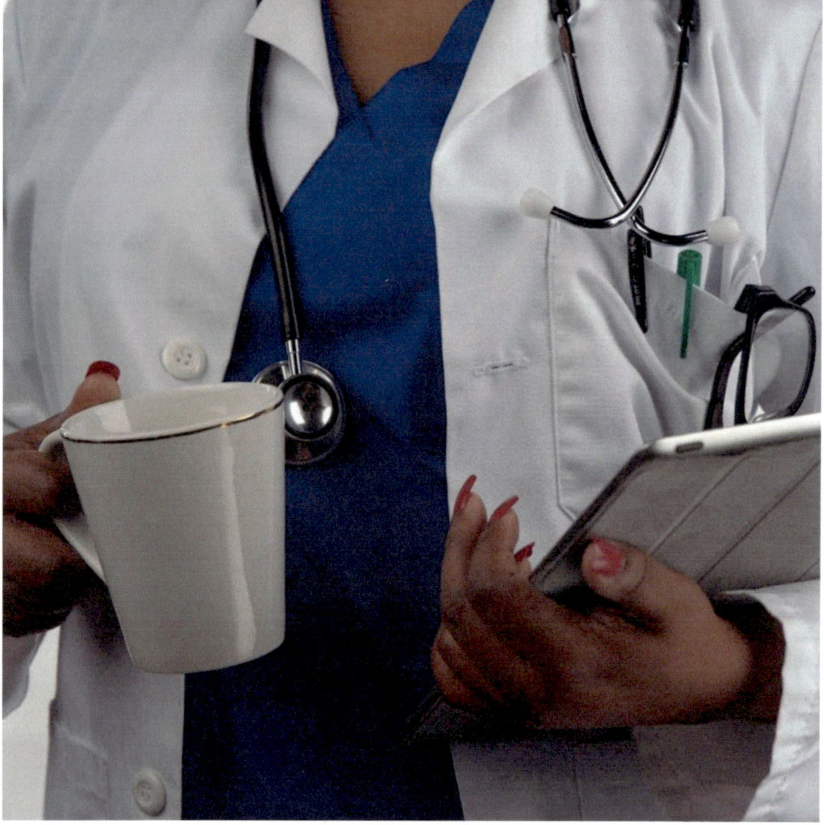

5

ERAS

(Electronic Residency Application Service)

A Parallel Plan

A parallel plan is like having a 'getting into residency' insurance policy. You don't really need to think about it until you need it. Have one from the onset.

Everyone should have a parallel plan in place. A parallel plan is a second specialty you will be as happy in as your first choice. *If you have made a running top three list of your specialty interest during the first couple of years of school*, then you already have parallel plan. You should make sure it is in place when you are creating the list of programs you will apply to. *Your list should include the specialty you are absolutely qualified for and a backup/dream specialty.* As you get interviews, you will begin to see where you are fitting in. If your dream is to be in Emergency Medicine but you only have three interviews; your back-up is Family Medicine, and you have ten interviews; you can now be realistic about how to structure both your rank list and your future plans to get into the emergency room. If you have done your research, you will know that it is not unusual to find Family Medicine physicians working in the emergency room. That's a parallel plan for getting where you want to be.

Filling Out the Application

Before filling out the ERAS application, my advice is to take the time to create a complete Curriculum Vita (CV). This will make filling out the application a whole lot simpler. You will be able copy and paste some of the information from your CV directly to the application. It will save you valuable time. The information on your CV will need to be placed in three major categories, -work experience, research experience, and volunteer experience. Remember to also list your publications, posters, presentations, abstracts, awards, and affiliations appropriately.

DO NOT leave the hobbies and interest section empty. Many an interview has revolved around commonalities found in the hobbies and interest section of the application. Here is something to consider: if you interviewed 25 candidates today and one had kayaking in common with you, whom would you remember? I will warn you however, not to lie. You *must* be able to intelligibly discuss the items on your list. For example, if you list cooking in your hobbies section, when asked 'what is your favorite item to cook?' your answer cannot be 'hummus' or 'salad'.

Take your time filling out the application. Be sure to fill-in all the requested information. Do not forget to release your USMLE score and register with NRMP.

Once your application has been completed, have someone that is not part of the process to review it for you. A classmate is not a viable option since they too have been viewing the application for long periods of time and may not be able to spot mistakes as readily as a new eye.

Lastly, print to pdf a copy of your application for later reference.

LoR's – What to keep in mind.

When I reviewed and uploaded letters of recommendations years ago, I came upon an interesting phenomenon. Students usually think they need to ask someone who knows them really well for a letter of recommendation. While that is true, I also found that letters from attending's they did not work with closely can be just as helpful.

Here is the reasoning. If you have worked closely with Dr. X for the past month or more, Dr. X eventually will have seen you when you came in a little late…, or before your morning coffee, or when you were tired-and your mood wasn't as great. Although not held against you, this knowledge affects, or as I like to say, '*colors*' Dr. X's writing about you. On the other hand, if Dr. Y only saw you for two weeks and every morning you were on time, in a good mood and fulfilled your requirements, this too, will affect or *'color'* Dr. Y's writing. If all, your recommender saw was an excellent student doctor, it is going to come across in their writing. If they saw the average student doctor, they happen to like, that will also come across in their writing. So, diversify in the types of people you ask for your letters of recommendation.

NOTE TO STUDENTS; when on rotations at home or away put your best foot forward at all times. You never know who is watching or talking; if it is the specialty of your choice, you should treat it as an audition.

You should also beware of situations where you do not get along with the resident but work well with the attending. Asking that attending for a letter is also a risk. Do not for one moment think that the attending has not spoken to the resident who has worked with you about your performance. Even worse do not think that the resident hasn't expressed how they feel about you to the attending.

I can't tell you how many times I have seen a great letter of recommendation that was spoiled with what I call the '*sandwich factor*'. The letter starts out with positive comments, there is one sentence mentioning a weakness and then the letter resumes to the pleasantries of 'I strongly recommend them'. These letters are not beneficial because what readers tend to remember is the outlier statement.

Pay attention to personalities on rotations and know who you are asking for your letters. If by chance, a letter writer asks you for a sample or template, *treat that as a gift*. You should then sit down and write yourself the best letter of recommendation ever. Remember, the more adjectives used to describe you and your working ability, the better and stronger the letter will be. Present that as your sample and hope that a close version of it becomes your letter of recommendation.

Here is a guide:

- Start by introducing the writer. Name, title, and organization.
- Tell how the writer knows the applicant; include a description of your relationship and length of time you have known them.
- State that you are pleased to write this letter for the applicant; state the applicant's full name.
- Use as many adjectives as you can when describing and assessing-academic achievements; the applicant's ability to work and communicate constructively with others.
- Describe characteristics, interests, research, special projects, coursework, and activities that demonstrate an interest in medicine or a particular specialty.
- Close by stating you are happy to support this candidate for the specialty of their choosing and how you can be reached: (contact info.).

Transcripts

Make sure your *transcript* is as up to date as possible when July rolls around. The transcript is uploaded by the institution. You do not control when or how it is uploaded. So do your part by making sure evaluations are completed, and grades are submitted and reflected on whatever system your school uses to allow you to view your grades.

Releasing the USMLE

Medical Students often debate the best time to release their USMLE scores. I have heard that if you have a good Step 1 score, then you should not release your Step 2 unless it is higher than your Step 1. Or, if you do not have a great Step 1 score, you should wait until your Step 2 scores come back before releasing both scores. I don't agree with any of that. If your Step score isn't great leaving it as the last thing a program director sees before deciding on your application may not be the best idea. Whether your score is good or bad waiting till the last possible moment to upload it may cost you interview offers.

Consider the fact that there are programs that will not offer an interview until you have a completed application package. Other programs will offer you an interview without it but will not rank you unless they get it. There are few programs that say they will rank you without it. You should always want to err on the side of caution by having your scores available. You do not want to look like you have something to hide. Ultimately those scores must be released, so go on and release them.

MSPE (Medical Student Performance Evaluation)

Your MSPE is usually constructed by the Office of Student Affairs. MSPE's differ as schools differ. It is an evaluation of the students' total performance in medical school.

It is my suggestion that you make an effort to know what is in your MSPE. Rules surrounding the MSPE vary from institution to institution. Find out what the rules are at your institution. Knowing what is in your MSPE is in your best interest. It is a document that will follow you well beyond fellowships. Therefore, if you are given the opportunity to contribute to any portion, you will need to do your best writing. If you are not able to contribute, make an appointment to view it or have a student copy sent to you. Make sure to check the accuracy of the factual data.

Third year evaluations from attending's are often included in MSPE's. If you have a problem with an evaluation, *after* the MSPE is written is *not* the time to challenge. Administrators have an absolute deadline to upload those letters. So, at *that* point you will become more of an annoyance. Staff members are no doubt pushing hard to meet the deadline. It is the exception that they will stop the process to accommodate you. To avoid such a situation, check your evaluations as they become available. If there is a problem with an evaluation, follow your institutions policies and guidelines to appeal it. File appeals *way* in advance so that your MSPE is complete and ready for upload.

Photo

I have seen everything from cropped group photos, selfies, passport photos, and no photo at all uploaded by students for ERAS. Please remember that this is a job application. I know that we are in the age of selfies but unless that program director is closer to your age, or older and very understanding it will not make a very good impression-so get a professional photo taken for ERAS. Think of it this way. If you have applied to thirty programs what are the chances of all thirty program directors being okay with your selfie? Now, what are the chances of all thirty of them being okay with a professional photo? I hope you've gotten my point. It is just better you err on the side of caution and be professional. If they want to see nonprofessional photos of you, they'll just search you on one of the social media sites. This leads me to this point. If there is something on your social media site that you don't want program directors to see such as you twerking at the Christmas party that was held off campus, then you should clean up your site way in advance of ERAS.

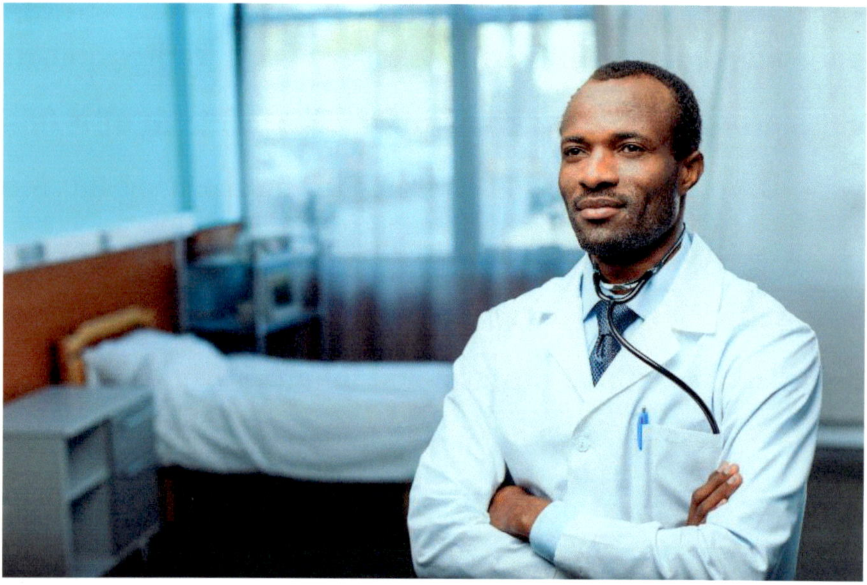

6

FOURTH YEAR

The timing of CS and CK

I believe that there is really no perfect time to take CS and CK… except when you're ready. Once January rolls around in your third year, the time clock starts ticking louder than ever in your head; and registering and finding a date takes priority. The specialty you choose will largely dictate the best time to take the test. The earlier you get the Clinical Skills (CS) test out of the way the better. Those results take longer to return than Clinical Knowledge (CK). Since CS is a very subjective test, if by some chance you do not pass, you will have time to retake it before submitting your ERAS application and going on interviews. *(Please note that as of 2020 the CS test is no longer a requirement. This may or may not be a permanent change.)* For CK take a pre-test before you schedule a date. It will let you know where your baseline is. Your results on the pre-test will give you an idea of what your study schedule should look like: lots of study time vs. pacing yourself. While there is no perfect time to take CS and CK there is such a thing as waiting till it's too late to take the test. Keep in mind that programs can begin ranking students as early as mid-January. You should take the test in time for your score to be available by then. You certainly wouldn't want to be placed on a pending or waiting list while those coveted rank spots disappear. It could certainly affect your ranking status with some programs.

You have gone through medical school with the goal of matching into a residency. Your best chances are for you to minimize all risks and maximize all chances at matching.

The Importance of September and October Deadlines

Please keep in mind that the September and October deadlines were put there for a reason.

September is the student's submission month. It is also when applications become available to programs. It is of course, in your best interest to have your application submitted by that deadline. However, an application can be submitted any time after the submission date.

October is the month for the MSPE's to be uploaded to the system. The upload of the MSPE is completed by the medical school. It is usually done by the Office of Student Affairs or your Student Affairs Dean. Keep in mind that since this is the last piece to complete the application process, you should also have completed uploading all the items needed by then. After the MSPE, programs tend to expect completed applications on the system.

Specialty Specifics

A few specialties require special planning to get positive results in the match process. Emergency Medicine (EM) is one such specialty. You will need at least one SLOE

(Standardized Letter of Evaluation) or SLOR (Standardized Letter of Recommendation) when applying, -two if possible. You can only get a valued SLOE/SLOR from a rotation that has an emergency medicine residency program. If your school does not have a residency program, you should apply for and do your EM rotations early, so that you can have a SLOE/SLOR uploaded before interviews are offered for the specialty. Interviews are usually offered around the beginning of November for EM. Most students are doing away rotations August thru November, which is why interviews don't really start coming till then. Remember there are exceptions to every rule, so having your documents ready early is a good idea.

Having a LoR (Letter of Recommendation) from another institution that is not your home institution looks good for Anesthesiology, Surgery and Orthopedic Surgery. Because program directors know students are still doing away rotations in the earlier months, interviews are offered in November and later, for those specialties as well.

Students in other specialties like Pediatrics, Internal Medicine, Psychiatry, Family Medicine, and Obstetrics and Gynecology can begin to get interviews by September. Have as much as possible of your application completed by then. Although students applying to these specialties are certainly open to doing away rotations, it is not necessary for obtaining interviews or matching.

With specialties like Dermatology, Radiation Oncology and Radiology, having research in the field is helpful and for some programs even necessary. These specialties are looking to see how strong your foundation in the field is.

Subspecialties and combination specialties are all competitive, so make sure you have a strong parallel plan in place when applying.

Interviews and the Interview Trail

After September, interviews start to go out. If you have not done one or two mock interviews over the summer months now is the time to get one done. I usually like to video-record mock interviews of students and play them back for students so they can see what I see. It's usually an eye-opening experience for them. They get a chance to see the details of who they are. Sometimes they even find out things about themselves that they didn't realize. It gives them a chance to put their best foot forward as they hit the interview trail or do online interviews.

Here are a few tips;

- ✓ ***Tip:*** *For online interviews make sure your background is not busy, untidy, or distracting.* I strongly suggest staging your background. Auto backgrounds can be distracting if every time you move it adjusts.

- ✓ ***Tip:*** *Be aware of how much you use your hands when you talk.* I do this a lot. I spent years doing sign language and interpreting so I tend to speak with my hands even when I am not signing. Some people do it without even knowing. If you find yourself doing it modify your behavior right away. Also, beware of little quirks about your communication that you may need to modify. Looking up at the ceiling while you are thinking, playing with your ear, wiping your face every other sentence, saying 'like' too much or cultural jargons like 'you know' are all things you should beware of. Doing a video of yourself during a mock interview is a good way to catch these things.

✓ ***Tip:*** *Be in control of your interview.* Many people go to interviews intending to be an open book. They think this will make people like them. Not so. There is something called being *too* open. Give only information that is requested and be relevant if giving additional information. Stay positive with your answers and do not be pushed into answering illegal questions. Questions that break both HIPPA and AAMC protocol. (Are you planning on getting married or having a baby? What other programs did you apply to?)

- ✓ **Tip:** *Learn how to give an answer without answering.* On the interview trail there will be times you come across people asking illegal questions. Never answer those questions outright. Here is an example: If you're asked; are you planning to have children? Your answer should be vague. Something like; *You never know what life has to offer.* And if they push, tell them; *That is a question I cannot answer at this time.* Learning to give an answer without answering the question is a skill you may want to get familiar with just in case you need to utilize it. Stay in control.

- ✓ **Tip:** *Be prepared for trick questions that are meant to throw you off your game.* Questions like…; what are some of the things you would change about medical school? Do not fall for this and go on a rant about all the things that are wrong at your institution. One of our students did just that. The interviewer called an old classmate who works at our institution. …who then called me. That year, even with *sixteen* interviews, the student did not match.

- ✓ ***Tip:*** *Choose to go a step further and answer questions differently; with a little more thought than usual.* Most people answer the question 'What are some of your strengths and weaknesses?' by giving two lists one of strengths and one of weaknesses. But think about it: a person's greatest strengths can also be their greatest weaknesses. If you are very organized, that is a great thing when organization is called for. But there are times-like at a family picnic, -when everyone just wants to relax. You become frustrated when your list of activities may not be needed. Those times your organizational skills may work against you... your strength become a weakness. Think a little beyond the norm in the way you answer questions. You will be remembered for it.

- ✓ ***Tip:*** *Pack light but pack a spare.* When traveling, be prepared for Murphy's Law: 'Anything that can go wrong will go wrong.' Pack interchangeable outfits; get mini containers for all your products; make copies of your important documents and store them in the pocket or lining of your suitcase; make sure you have directions to *everywhere*. Put every contingency that you can think of in place.

- ✓ ***Tip:*** *Do not turn down interviews unless there is an absolute conflict, or you have reached your max financially*. Keep in mind that the more programs you can list on your rank list the better for you in terms of matching. Consider the fact that matching to the tenth program on your rank list is better than not matching and having to SOAP. Also, matching at a program that is less than ideal is better than not matching.

When making plans for the interview trail, some students may choose not to go to the pre-interview dinner. Although it is a matter of choice you should highly consider going. The pre-interview is where you network, find out more about the program, and decide if you fit in. If you attend the pre-interview dinner and make a connection with someone, it may help in securing a spot. On the other hand, if you attend and do not connect with anyone, it will help you determine just where that program will rank.

Getting Your Schedule and Travel Plans in Order

Students are often surprised at how easy it is to get their schedules to line up in a way that keeps them from running back and forth; from coast to coast. If you are on a student's budget, this will save you a lot of time and money. Especially if you are wanting to match on the opposite coast. If you can plan your fourth-year schedule, it just makes sense to cluster, all your activity on one coast at a time.

Booking Travel

When you start to receive interview offers having a calendar is super important. You will need to make sure there are no conflicts when setting up interviews. When booking travel, if being cost-effective is important, consider all forms of travel, -rental, bus, train and plane. This is also the time when having a 'miles for spending' credit card comes in handy. If you are going to own a credit card before entering medical school, a 'miles for spending' credit card from an airline is a good idea. With all the spending you do in medical school, the miles are bound to add up and fourth year is when you can cash those miles in for free air fare to some of your interviews.

Please note: As of 2020, the year of COVID-19, interviews will be done online. You can keep these tips in mind however, for when things get back to normal.

The Importance of a Bucket List

You have just spent the last three and a half years with

your head buried (most of the time) in books and staring at computer screens. By the time interviews are winding down you will have more spare time on your hands than you have had in the last couple of years. Remember all this free time is about to be taken away again with the beginning of intern year. I always suggest to students that they create a bucket list of things they would like to do so that they can jumpstart their social life once again. No need to spend all of January and February obsessing about the rank list. Go out and have some fun, so that you can clear your mind and focus on what you really want your life in residency to be like.

Interviewing the Program

You should interview programs in the same way as they are interviewing you. Go to the pre-interview dinner if possible. Question the residents about how they spend their free time. Evaluate whether individuals there are happy and assess how you will fit in with them.

Remember programs create an environment for applicants. It is very easy to get caught up in the ‘I want to be liked’ mindset-so much so that you miss the little clues that will allow you to make proper decisions. I can’t tell you how many times students, who have ended up unmatched look at me with tears in their eyes and say, ‘but they said they were going to rank me’. These are the students who got caught up in the ‘I want to be liked’ mindset. They spend their time on the interview trying to impress, and do not take time to evaluate their surroundings or the people they encounter.

Do a second look if possible. When you visit the second time, ask questions. Try to find out what the workplace is like. Talk to individuals outside the interview process; find out how things run on an everyday basis. Speak to nurses, physician assistants, and janitors to get an idea of how they feel about the institution they are working for. You will want to know how things feel *outside* of the interview atmosphere that was created. Ask about quality of life and morale in the workplace. Inquire about duty hours and efficiency of systems. Identify the people who really like their jobs, because those are the ones you will want to have as mentors.

This will give you the ability to better asses the program and help you to create your rank list.

Keep in mind that when you go to an interview, programs know that you hold all the cards in the process, and they want the advantage. The way they get the advantage is to make sure every student who leaves the interview will want to put them first on their rank list. That way no matter who the programs choose for their rank list, they will be sure to get their choice of students. That is why they create what I call the interview bubble. It is an 'everyone is happy, we all want you, and all is well with the world' environment that happens only on interview days. Programs don't want to end up with unfilled positions. That only means they will have to spend more time flipping through applications in the SOAP-and programs do not want to be in the SOAP any more than you do. The SOAP is when they hold all the cards. Since you do not want to end up there, do your best in interviewing programs. It will help you to better make choices ranking your programs.

NOTE: The AAMC has an app called The MATCH PRISM that can help you track and rate each program.

You will want to evaluate what is important to you and consider those things. Here is a list of things to consider when in search of a program:

- Quality Mentorship
- Didactics
- Adequate Research
- Friendly residence/great team
- Case Variety
- A Program Director and Chair that communicates effectively
- Rotating at varying hospitals
- Good hospital facility
- Effective teaching, feedback, and direction
- A comfortable environment

- Happy staff/ resident wellness
- Consider serviced demographic and volume
- Program fellowship availability
- Ability to pursue another degree
- Residents' diversity
- Affordability of the city
- In house patient information system
- Time off
- Pay scale
- Prep time for boards

This is just a partial list of things you should think about when considering a program. My suggestion is that you put it in order of priority according to what is important to you.

Creating Your Rank List

The rank list is something students are known to toil over and study as if it was a STEP test. I suggest you go back to thinking about what will make you happy and make your choices based on that principle. Do not waste time trying to figure out who will choose you or how the algorithm works. Decide your rank list based on solid principles-which program were you most comfortable with, which residents were genuinely happy, which program director seemed easiest to talk to or have a discussion with. Think about what you really want and make your list based on that.

It is not a great idea to exclude programs you have interviewed with off your rank list. The question you should ask yourself is 'Would I rather SOAP or work at that program?'

7

OTHER CONCERNS

I'm Engaged, Now What?

Yes, you can plan a wedding and be in medical school. The key is to organize, organize, organize. Did I say organize? You will also need to freshen up your delegating skills.

I tend to suggest getting a bridal book as soon as you can. That will give you a list of what needs to be done. This will open the way for you to set a budget. Once that is done your next choice is to either get a wedding planner or decide who is going to be part of your wedding team. Then plan a weekend with your boo to make choices about basics like colors, numbers, and places. Once those things have been decided, delegate to-do list items with your wedding team or your planner. Here is an example of what I mean; you've decided that you want to have your wedding in Denver. You don't have time to research a location. Tell your planner or your team you need help finding a location. The suggestions will come pouring in and all you'll have to do is choose. You can do this for everything and keep friends and family happy by having them feel included in the planning of your special day. If done correctly, you'll be able to focus on school; when wedding issues arise, it will just be a matter of making a choice and moving on.

What date you set is up to you. No time is a 'best time' during medical school, but keep in mind that friends and family will already be in town around white coat/match week and graduation.

I'm Pregnant, Now What?

Every female handle getting pregnant in medical school differently. Some decide to take a year off. Some slow down their schedule and graduate off cycle in June or December. Then there are others who handle it as a boss and stay on schedule and graduate on time. No matter what you choose, be at peace with your decision and seek as much support as possible.

It is certainly not necessary for you to quit medical school because you are pregnant, and no-your medical career has not ended. If you decide to continue, it will mean that you will need to be super organized. If you take the year off, enjoy your time off, stay healthy, and be prepared to hit the ground running when you return. It will require you going from zero to sixty in record time. If, on the other hand, you decide to slow things down and graduate off schedule, go at your own pace and do not let *anyone* rush you. Keep in mind that your classmates will now be ahead of you, so you may not have them as study partners or to guide you as you progress. Make sure to handle yourself professionally as you request time off or reschedule exams. Do not expect anyone to be understanding of your plight but remember to be very grateful when they are. Try to work within the rules and *know* what the rules are.

Some schools will work with you and others will not. Know what you are dealing with and make the best decisions for yourself based on the cards you've been dealt.

A Family Member Has Died

There are so many things students seek my advice on besides academics; this happens to be one of them. I feel that the least number of words uttered tends to go further. After giving my condolences, I have a pdf that I send students. It has all the details needed to cover a funeral. There are suggestions listed for every phase of the process, and I remind them of the power of delegating tasks to get things done. What I hear from students later is that it empowered them to help where they could and made the process smoother and more efficient. Even if their contribution were to forward the document to a family member who was taking care of things, it made them feel like they were part of the process.

Getting Back into Medical School, After a Dismissal

If you have been dismissed from medical school for not passing courses, and you intend to re-apply, you will need to do a couple of things:

- ✓ First, identify what happened so you can fix it; show you know what went wrong, and that it will not happen again.
- ✓ Second, you will need to take coursework in the same subject areas you failed; it will show you've strengthened your foundational knowledge in that area.
- ✓ Finally, create a plan that shows how you will avoid repeating the same mistakes you made the first time.

Writing an Appeal

When writing an appeal letter do not do a 'brain dump'. That is when you just tell how you feel about what has happened and ask for a different result. Writing a letter like that does not give any helpful information; it can do more harm than good if the reader does not agree with you.

Come to terms with why you need to write the appeal letter in the first place. Make a list of the facts; make a list of your opinions/rebuttal. Start out with all the facts followed by your opinion/rebuttal.

Be specific and concise. Be chronological in expressing what has happened, why it has happened, and what you plan on doing about it.

Should I Take a Year Off for Research or a Fellowship?

If you will be applying to a specialty where research is needed, taking a year off to do research can help. If that is your choice, make sure that you do research with a leading or notable name in the specialty. If you are taking a year off for a fellowship, make sure it is in the specialty you will be applying to. At the end of your year off, request letters of recommendation from those you have worked with during that year.

Between third and fourth year is the best time to take off. That way you can refresh your clinical skills during your fourth-year clinical rotations and before starting your intern year.

If you are not a competitive candidate for a specialty, research will not make you more competitive. I have seen it time and time again. Students that are not competitive for a specialty take time off and do research-thinking it will make them a better candidate. They end up unmatched and needing to SOAP or getting stuck in prelim land. It is always good to have research experience, but if you take that year off to do research, make sure to have a parallel plan.

Networking is the name of the game during your year off. Meet as many individuals in the field as you can and be sure to let them know that you will be applying in the upcoming year. That way, if your name or application comes across their desk, it will be in your favor.

I'm Having Trouble with my USMLE's

Much of the same advice I gave in studying for Step 1 applies here. If, however, you are still not getting good scores on your practice tests, you should get tested to make sure you do not learn differently. I have found that there are students who make it all the way to medical school not knowing they have been compensating-at a high-level for learning differently. Because of the volume of information that must be learned, the length of time needed to stay focused, learning issues tend to become more evident. Now, are there students who just can't cut it? Yes, but you owe it to yourself to find out if there isn't an underlying reason/s your score isn't where you want there to be.

If there is a problem, you should seek help right away. Forget about stigmas. You have invested way too much in your career to stop now.

Bulling by Peers on Rotations

Document as much as possible; by using emails to clarify disagreements with your peers. Then follow the chain of command and put your issues in writing via email. Be chronological about the details. State clearly how you are feeling about the situation and ask for definite resolutions. When going up the chain of command does not work, seek help from the honor council or ethics board.

Sitting back and allowing others to get away with unfair treatment, whether to you or someone else, is being an active participant in their action. It empowers them to ill-treat the next person… and the next… and the next…. It is especially disheartening when this behavior is being perpetrated by doctors or student doctors. Eventually such behavior will spill over into the way they treat patients. Do everything you can to resolve the situations.

It is my opinion that mean and unhappy doctors hurt more than they heal. I, for one DO NOT tolerate such behavior.

I Did Not Match, Now What?

If you did not match in the main match, STOP! Put everything else on pause and focus on preparing for the SOAP. There will be time LATER to try and figure out what happened. There will be time LATER to feel disappointed, cry, explain to loved ones, and deal with classmates.

Preparing for the SOAP is an emotionally draining experience. Just seeing students go through it is emotionally draining for me. Here is a rundown of the day; I'm going to leave out times as they are subject to change but here is the general order:

First, you get an email that says you, are SOAP eligible.

- This is not telling you that you will be in the SOAP. It is simply giving you notice that you are eligible to participate.

A few hours later you receive a second email telling you one of three things:

❖ You have successfully matched.

This means you're fine. You can go celebrate. Please remember to be mindful of those not celebrating.

❖ You have partially matched.

This means one of two things. You have either matched for an advanced spot but not a preliminary spot or have matched for a preliminary spot but not an advanced spot. If this is the case, you will need to prepare to SOAP.

❖ You did not match.

This is when everything stops; you need to focus on your parallel plan. Although negative feelings will overwhelm you, do not waste time with them. Hit the PAUSE button on your negative feelings. You NEED to prepare for SOAP, and if you match in the SOAP, you will not need to express those feelings.

Within a few hours the SOAP will begin.

Here are a few suggestions as you prepare:

- Find a friend or an advisor to help you through this process. I know you think you can handle it by yourself; I know you don't really want to see anyone right now, but remember-isolation is *not* your friend at this moment.

- Gain access to two screens or a screen big enough to open two windows side by side. This will make the process easier as you will need to go back and forth between the ERAS and NRMP website. Having ERAS stationary on one and NRMP stationary on the other will save you time on loading. It will also save you aggravation on going back and forth using one screen.

- Have a friend help you do a little research on the programs that are available.

- Have a blazer nearby just in case you get an online

interview via facetime, skype or some other online platform.

Once you have submitted your first set of applications in the system, find something to do. Just sitting around waiting can be emotional torture. Keep your phone or tablet with you and do something. There is a day-and-a-half wait time till offers are posted. Do something, anything or emotional breakdown will occur. Remember to keep those negative feelings on PAUSE. You need to stay focused for interviews, and the second round.

On the last day of the SOAP a final list of unfilled positions is posted. Make note of the positions that are still unfilled so that you can contact those programs after the SOAP has officially ended. If after the SOAP has ended, you still don't have a position, you can officially hit UNPAUSE on the negative feelings; purge your emotions, and deal with family, friends and classmates. Watching classmates celebrate on match day will be especially hard, so do prepare emotionally. Although tempting, isolation is still not your friend. When asked 'where did you match?' I suggest you have a planned answer like "I'm still looking. If you know of any place or anyone, I should contact please let me know.' Now I know it's hard, but the more individuals that know you're still looking the better chances you have that someone can make a call or speak on your behalf.

I have had a student who did not match, and subsequently asked their church to pray for them. Because there were a few doctors in the audience one made a call to a classmate whose program happened to have one open spot. That classmate then spoke to their department Chair, and the student had a job by the end of the week. Once again, I know it is hard, but isolation is *not* your friend.

Post SOAP: Still Unmatched.

- Create a file for yourself that contains: (1.) any *letters of recommendation* you may have, (2.) a student copy of your *MSPE*, (3.) a copy of your *medical school transcript*, (4.) a copy of your *USMLE* Step scores (1 & 2 CK and CS), (5.) your *CV or ERAS application*, and (6.) *personal statement.*

- Find every business card from every program director you may have gotten one from on the interview trail. Keep them handy.

After the SOAP you can begin to contact programs and show interest in their unfilled positions. Check www.findaresident.com or any other website you may know of for positions. REMEMBER: isolation is still not your friend. Reach out to everyone; let them know you are looking for a position. This is when classmates and upper-class mentors can come in handy. Get a few friends to help you look for unfilled positions or to make calls on your behalf. Call up alumni, physician friends, or even physician family members to keep an eye out on your behalf. The larger your network, the better chance you have of getting a position before July 1. So put embarrassment, shyness, and ego on the side and build a network.

COVID-19

As if individuals in the medical field did not have enough to worry about, 2020 rolled around and Covid-19 changed everything. For the medical student, here are some of the changes brought about.

- *The due dates for ERAS have changed.* Yes, you have a little more time, but do not let time slip away and put you in a rush to get things done.

- *The interview process will be held online.* That means you should find a spot early, one that you will use to do interviews. Stage the area to be interview ready by making sure your background is not too busy, or totally empty. Put conversational pieces, awards or even research posters in your background to make it interesting. Make sure you have a strong

Wi-Fi signal. Since you will be doing most things online, invest a bit of money for proper Wi-Fi.

- *Clinical Skills (CS) has been canceled*; for now.

- *Most programs are having an online open house.* Make sure you attend; this is how you will get to know Program Directors and Chairmen. It is also a time to ask questions so you can get to know more about the program.

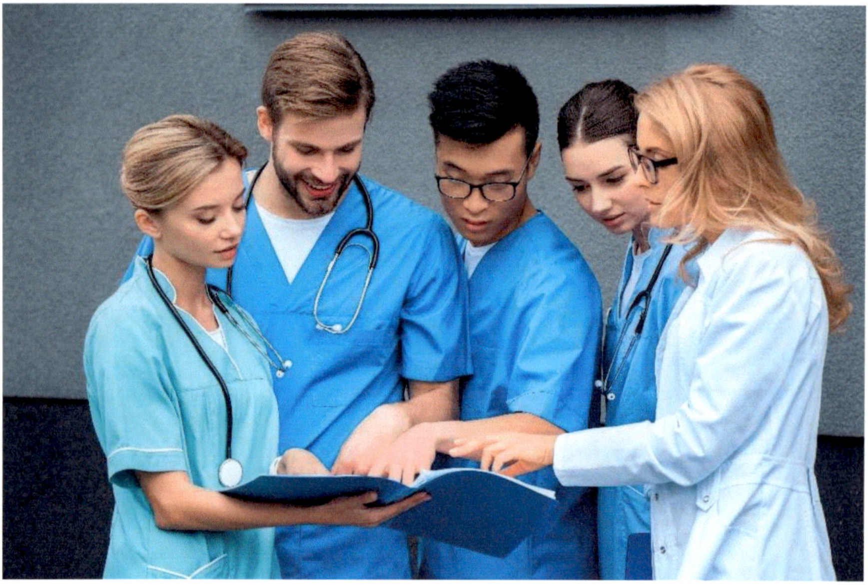

8

FIRST YEAR RESIDENTS

I Don't Like Where I Matched, What Do I Do?

Remember that the match is a contract; know about and read your contract carefully.

Keep in mind that you do not have much time after the match ends before the re-application cycle for the next year begins. Each ERAS administrator decides when to start the process for the following year. For now, you can simply transfer your application from one year to another. You will need to send out requests for letters of recommendation and reload all documentation to the system. Also, keep a close eye on your schedule for the coming year in residency, as you will need to schedule interviews in the fall. You may need to sacrifice your vacation time to do interviews.

Do not blindside your program director by applying without their knowledge. They will not like the idea that they have made an investment in choosing you for their program, and you are essentially jumping ship. Therefore, you may need to be strategic about when you have that conversation-but *have* the conversation. You will also need a letter of recommendation from your program director to move from one program to another. I can't tell you enough just how big a risk that is. Blindsiding your program director is a *bad* idea.

If you are going to try to transfer, you can only do so a certain number of days after your official start date, based on current contracts. Contracts can change from year to year. Read your contract.

I Don't Like This Specialty Anymore

If you find yourself unhappy during your first year, ask yourself this question: 'In four years would I rather be an unhappy chief or a happy resident?' It's one year. You are going to be a physician for the rest of your life. Invest the time in yourself and re-apply. Remember happy doctors save lives, unhappy doctors can cost you your life. Which do you want to be? Consider this advice; do what will make you happy.

Applying to ERAS Again

If you are applying to ERAS for the following year, remember the next cycle starts in April two weeks after you receive your initial match results. You will need to get as much done as possible before you begin intern year. Contact your ERAS administrator to find out if there are any changes to the process. Request a token.

I'm Being Asked to Leave My Program

First, try to regroup and figure out why you are being asked to leave. Sometimes it is because there is a personality conflict. Other times it is because you cannot keep up with the demands of the institution. Try to transfer or re-apply before your exit date. If it is before year two has ended, try to pass Step 3 before you leave.

If it is for reasons such as you fell sick or got pregnant seek legal advice.

No matter what the reasons, know your rights; make sure to get a copy of your personnel file before you leave.

9

INTERNATIONAL STUDENTS

US Senior Internationals

International students who have gone to school in the US are a little different from internationals that are abroad. Since you are already in the US, paperwork and visas do not have to be filed to come here. Be sure however, to get your additional paperwork done early. This makes your transition to residency easier. However, when you are making the list of schools you will apply to, you will need to put in a little extra work.

You should research programs in your specialty that offer visas. These programs can be your first pool of programs. Your second pool of programs should be schools that do not state whether they do visas or not. The only programs you should exclude are the ones that expressly state they do not accept visas.

Internationals from Abroad

One of the reasons American seniors who have not matched can still snag a residency spot in June, is because paperwork can sometimes not come through in time for internationals from abroad to start in July. From my limited experience things tend to move a little slower abroad then they do here in the U.S. Therefore, make sure to fill out your paperwork in a timely manner and follow up on it.

You do not have the luxury of starting this process in August. I get third year American students started on ERAS in January so that they can pace themselves and be ready in September. If you are an international student, you should start in November of the year before the cycle begins by getting the list of what you will need to do. Start the process during your down time in December by doing your CV and personal statement. This will get you ready for VSAS/VSLO. Apply to VSAS/VSLO in January and file the paperwork for necessary visas to travel.

When you travel for your rotation networking is the name of the game. If you can, time your travel to sync with conventions or conferences in your specialty. Bring business cards with you and try to meet as many program directors as possible. You should try to visit program directors from other institutions in the area.

Please note: As of 2020, the year of COVID-19, this can all be done online.

Visa Status

Information is power. Do not just sit back and rely on the hospital to do everything when it comes to getting your visa. Know which visa you will be applying for and know what the process is to get it. Know what the hospital protocol is for getting it and who will facilitate the process. You should also know what you will need to do and who you will need to contact to make sure the process is on track.

How to Create My List of Programs

International students should consider creating their list of prospective programs in a way that can maximize their chances of matching. Here are a few suggestions:

- ✓ Don't just look for programs that state they offer visas, although you will want to know specifically which ones *do* so you can apply to those first. They should not be the only ones you apply to. If a program does not give a statement about visas, apply, because if you get an interview and they like you, they will accept you.

- ✓ Do look for programs that state they DO NOT offer visas and do not waste money on those.

- ✓ Make sure you know what paperwork will be required from a program if you are accepted.

- ✓ Do not just leave it up to the program to do everything. Find out how and in what way you can contribute to the process and follow up with *everything*.

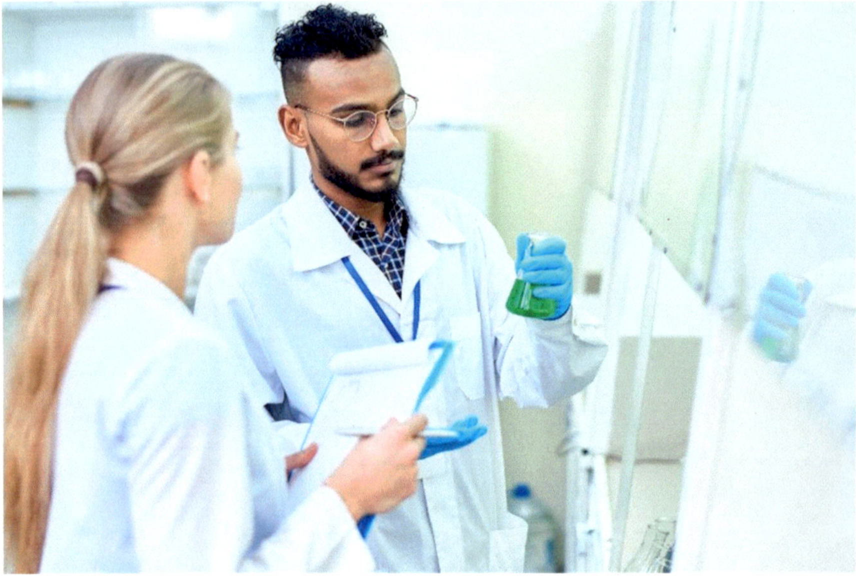

10

OTHER MATCHES

Applying to the Canadian Match, the Military Match & the San Francisco Match

The Canadian Match (CARMS), the Military Match (MODS) and the San Francisco Match (SF Match) are different from ERAS. Their open and close dates are also different. Therefore, if you are applying, find out what the due dates are and be mindful of them.

Be sure to go online and find out what is required from you. Each match has a portal, for the uploading of documents. Be sure to remind the dean's office administrator to do your upload before due dates. So far, each match tries to keep their due dates for the MSPE the same as ERAS.

The SF and Military match dates are earliest, and the

results are available in December.

I suggest that even though you are applying to these matches you should apply to ERAS as a backup.

Please Note: *Because of COVID-19 travel advice may not be as applicable this year but do keep it in mind for when things get back to normal.*

11

WHY DID I WRITE THIS BOOK?

I have been asked on several occasions 'Leiza, why aren't you a medical doctor?' Here is my short answer. I am a very spiritually minded person; I believe being a medical doctor is a calling, although I am certainly capable of doing so, it is not my calling. Teaching is.

Many situations in my life have reverberated that fact. The sight of even my own blood at times can cause nausea. As a child, I have always suffered from "white coat syndrome". I was well into my twenties before I became calm enough to go to a doctor without tears being involved. The stories of my hysteria as a child when seeing a doctor, although funny to others, still aren't funny to me. I am completely convinced that the hospital setting is not for me.

What I do remember, however, is the disposition of that first doctor who was able to calm me. He was happy, he was reassuring, and he was willing to wait until I was ready to receive that needle. I was not just another number passing through. He told me step by step what he was about to do, and most of all, he changed my perspective. I remember thinking that I wish there were more doctors like him.

I kept him as my doctor for the next eight years. Eventually I needed to leave where I lived and move to another city. Feeling how I did about most doctors at the time, the medical school was not my first choice of where to work. Having help with my job search, the offer came from where I was not expecting. I was surprised to receive an offer to work at a medical school. If I had a rank list it would have been at the bottom of the list. But the job pretty much fell in my lap, and I needed to work.

The job of an administrative assistant in the Deans office at that medical school was supposed to be a pit stop in my life's plan of becoming an elementary school teacher. Teaching, -that was my gift- and that is what I had been doing up 'till' then. I remember walking into the College of Medicine on my first day thinking 'One year, just one year. I'm out of here as soon as I can.' As it turns out, God had other plans for my life.

After my year in the Dean's office, I was ready to go. I had enough of sitting behind a desk, pushing paperwork, and answering calls. The Dean at the time, however, decided to move me to the job of Student Affairs Program Coordinator. I had no idea what the role entailed at the time. After talking to the Associate Dean of Student Affairs-my new boss-about what was required of me, I knew I could handle the tasks I was given, but I was curious about what the overall goal of the office was. So, I started to research, and I paid attention to the everyday details. What I learned was that only about seventy percent of all students who went through this medical school became actual doctors. Hmmm, why was that? I discovered that the task I was given of managing the

Deans Workstation (DWS) for ERAS had something to do with it. After speaking to a few of the students, I realized that they knew even less about the process than I did. *Well, no wonder* so many of them were not successful! They simply did not know what they were doing. My personality is not one that would just go with the flow. Whatever I did, or was a part of, needed to be successful.

I wanted to be educated enough to give students the information they needed about the process. Bit by bit I realized what the flaws were in their application process. As I spoke to program directors and went to AAMC meetings, I became more familiar with the process. I spoke with other DWS managers and to students from other schools, and with each year that went by, I adjusted our process and educated students about what was needed. The match rate where I worked eventually rose to ninety-five percent.

Please note that getting to ninety-five percent was not the result of just me. Many individuals worked to help us get to that number. However, in focusing on my role in the process, I became re-acquainted with the fact that knowledge is power. By educating students to the process, providing resources, advisors, and making them knowledgeable about what was expected of them, rates rose.

Students are still as clueless about this process in their third year as they were when I first started years ago. They simply do not have time to invest before it's required. I see a clear difference in the ones who are advised and the ones who are not. What I have also discovered is that students who come in earlier tend to go through this process less stressed, and with better results.

This has led me to thinking *'what if students came into medical school with the end game in mind and a clear path to follow? What if they were educated about the details and nuances of the process?'* This would give even underprivileged students who enter medical school a fair chance at finishing with the best of the bunch.

So here it is, the nuances of going through medical school and into residency. You or other administrators may not agree with everything that is said here. Fact is that a bit of it may seem a little unorthodox. But like I tell my students, take the advice that can benefit you and leave the rest. Some part of this book will make your medical school journey a little less stressful, and some parts simply will not apply to you.

Knowledge is power and it is also half the battle. Good luck in your endeavors.

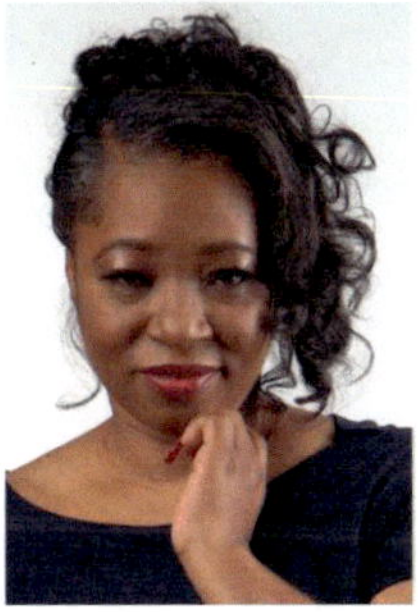

ABOUT THE AUTHOR

Leiza O'Neil has worked in academia for the past twenty-eight years. She started working as a Career Development Counselor during summers for the NYC Board of Education Metro Guide System in 1990. There she distributed information and counseled college-bound high school students about application requirements, overnight visits, and financial aid information. She then went on to work as a teacher's aide and later as a computer teacher and technician. She became a computer consultant, setting up computer labs for both private and public schools. She was also consulted to develop an elementary school computer lab curriculum. The curriculum she developed was widely used across the private elementary school sector in New York City. Being Microsoft and Network Certified, she was later tapped as a consultant to work as a visiting Instructor at Adelphi University, teaching the Microsoft Suite to welfare recipients in a federally funded program. The following year, she left Adelphi University to work at Howard University College of Medicine as an administrative assistant in the Office of the Dean.

At Howard University Ms. O'Neil has worked with the HR Director maintaining the HR Microsoft Access database; she also worked as the coordinator for the College-Wide Appointment, Promotions and Tenure Committee. She then transitioned to the being the Student Affairs Program Coordinator. In that capacity she has coordinated residency fairs, managed over 50 interest groups, organizations, anniversary celebrations, wellness programs, developmental workshops, honors and oath ceremonies, long and short white coat ceremonies, career nights and freshman orientation. She has sat on the HUCOM Liaison Committee on Medical Education (LCME), the National Medical Association (NMA) Convention Planning Committee, and both the Howard

University 140th and 150th Anniversary Planning Committee. She was also a presenter for the Writing Personal Statements and CV's Workshop at the Student National Medical Association 50th Anniversary Convention. Ms. O'Neil's focus, however, has been working with students as the Program Coordinator for the Electronic Residency Application Service. In that capacity she has worked diligently to help students with all aspects of the process, to ensure that they match into residency. Since working as the Student Affairs Program Coordinator, the match rate has risen over 20 points. With diligent work and perseverance, the match rate is consistently on the rise. For those who would have her, getting help with every aspect of the application process, including but not limited to CV's, personal statements, mock interviews, scheduling, Visiting Student Application Service (VSAS), now known as Visiting Student Learning Opportunities (VSLO), and personal issues are all part of her everyday tasks. The expertise that she has gained over the years is what she hopes to share with hopeful medical students all over this country who may need a little extra help or direction in getting into residency.

Made in the USA
Las Vegas, NV
04 November 2026

57426981R00083